THE
POWER
TO BE WELL

*How to live well
with diabetes*

To Sheila

CATHERINE FESTE
Award-winning author and speaker

Be well !

Cathy Feste

Cover design and composition,
Joni McPherson
Editor, Sherrye Landrum
Printer, SPS Publications

ISBN 1-881099-52-0

This book is derived from the award-winning, EMPOWERMENT: A Personal Path to Responsible Self-Care program developed by Catherine Feste and evaluated in a randomized, controlled trial at the University of Michigan with people who have diabetes. Outcomes included a clinically significant improvement in A1c, improved attitudes and increased self-efficacy. *Diabetes Care,* July, 1995.

Dedication

With admiration and gratitude this book
is lovingly dedicated to my father-in-law
and mother-in-law, Chris and Ruth Feste.
Their lives have been an inspiring
example of the power to be well.

Contents

Preface vi

Foreword xi

Acknowledgments xiv

Introduction 1

Personal Goals: Set Your Own 4

Optimism: The Philosophy and
Practice of Problem Solving 21

Wisdom: How to Tap Yours 39

Energy: Renew Through Stress
Management 49

Resilience: Build with Reflection . . . 64

End Notes 78

Preface

Why do some people do well when confronted with challenges? That question has guided my life's work. My response is, "Because they are healthy people."

Today we use the word *empowerment* to describe the process we go through in solving problems or achieving goals, in which we access and use psychological, social, emotional, and spiritual resources.

People with a chronic disease like diabetes need to understand the differences between the empowerment model in healthcare and patient education and the compliance-based model. For many years patients were simply told what to do (take this medication; follow this diet) and were expected to comply (do exactly as they were told). The compliance model does not take into account the fact that people make their own choices. But we do. And our choices are based on our values, goals, needs, and problems as *human beings*.

In the empowerment model, we are encouraged to focus on our own lives. We are aware of diabetes and its requirements, but we are devoted to the pursuit of a fulfilling life. This does not mean we ignore diabetes. It means we have both life goals and goals for managing diabetes.

In the compliance model, the power belongs to the health professionals. In the empowerment model, the power is shared between patients and health professionals. No patient is ever called "non-compliant" because the focus is on becoming aware, personal responsibility, informed choices, and quality of life. A health professional is a technical advisor who shares knowledge about diabetes. You are the expert on your own life. You are no longer a passive member of the team who simply takes orders. You make informed choices and decisions for your own health, and you have the responsibility to carry out those decisions.

The compliance model focuses on problems. Health insurance companies promote this because most require the diagnosis of a problem to cover a clinic visit. Empowerment is concerned with preventing problems. Empowerment education, with its focus on the health of the whole person, should be offered to every person diagnosed with diabetes (or any chronic disease that is largely patient-managed). Empowerment education promotes life skills like coping and problem solving and encourages professional counseling and peer counseling.

Are you wondering why so few people are empowered? Many are overwhelmed with life challenges or have not yet learned that they have other options. Hopelessness becomes the greatest foe. But empowerment education gives you a feeling of being in control. You are on the leading edge of the paradigm shift from the compliance model to the empowerment approach. It will take time to overcome the inertia to change and bad habits. But remember this: The process of empowering ourselves never ends. We will always have new goals, new problems, new solutions. These goals and problems lead us to new growth and a better connection to our own power. The professional members of the American Association of Diabetes Educators are aware and trained in the empowerment model. They can assist you in the process of becoming and staying empowered. To find a diabetes educator in your area, call: 1-800-832-6874.

Our responsibility, as people who have diabetes, is to fully engage in the process of empowering ourselves. The process is outlined in this book: **Personal** awareness leads to better choices. **Optimism** provides a hopeful, helpful frame of mind for problem solving. **Wisdom** informs us about the choices that are most meaningful to us. **Energy** renewal is vital because this process is wearying. **Resilience** helps us to bounce back when life lays us flat. Taken all together we have: **POWER**.

*Look to this day for it is the life of
Life.*

*In its brief course lie all the
verities and realities of existence.*

*For yesterday is but a dream and
tomorrow is only a vision,*

*But today, well-lived, makes every
yesterday a dream of happiness*

And every tomorrow a vision of hope.

Look well, therefore, to today.

It is the life of Life.

—KALIDASA

Foreword

Living well with diabetes is a challenge. It requires discipline, persistence, courage, wisdom, faith, and optimism. In this book, my dear friend, Cathy, pulls together her many years of living well with diabetes and helps to motivate you with the golden nuggets of her faith, outlook, optimism and experience and encourages you to find *your* motivation to be well.

Since I was diagnosed with diabetes in 1968 and thereafter, I have found that a lot of people freely give both solicited and unsolicited advice about diabetes and how to manage it. Most folks are well-intentioned, and I am okay with receiving their offer of help. In truth, however, I have received both practical and impractical advice, motivational encouragement, pessimistic doom and gloom, and sometimes an espoused philosophy that allowed me to understand they didn't have a clue what it is like to actually live with this disease! Much of it did not stick with me in the early years, but some things did. And those pithy thoughts that did stick, molded my personal philosophy of care. Here are a few examples of those thoughts that have molded me and my own diabetes management.

When life deals out lemons, make lemonade.
– poster in blood-drawing laboratory

Know your enemy. – my uncle and physician, Robert Kleinschmidt, MD

That which does not break me will serve to make me stronger. – Friedrich Nietzsche

You get the bear or the bear gets you.
– folk wisdom

Do your best! – my mom

How do we do it? The hard way! – my kids (who liked short-cuts!)

I can do all things through Christ who strengthens me. – Philippians 4:13

With wisdom, humor and common sense, Cathy pulls from literature, anecdotes, and stories to give us perspective on managing diabetes. After thinking about what Cathy has written here, you may find some nuggets that will stick with you and mold your own philosophy of self care. Cathy has woven her experience in motivation, storytelling and diabetes management to give you some wonderful insights. May your reflections give you wisdom.

Jean Betschart Roemer
CRNP, MN, MSN, CDE

Acknowledgments

The Menninger Foundation's Center for Applied Behavioral Sciences provided great professional grounding. I am thankful for their vision and their use of story, cartoons, music and humor to help people see the human side of behavior in *Toward Understanding Human Behavior and Motivation*.

Herb Benson, MD, and his gifted staff at Harvard Medical School's Mind/Body Institute, provided wonderful nourishment in the classes I took with them: *Healing & Spirituality and Mind/Body Training in Positive Psychology*.

The National Storytelling Network has been an important source of education and leadership. Thanks especially to mentors Allison Cox, Gail Rosen and Laura Simms.

The American Association of Diabetes Educators (AADE) continues to be my professional family. After 30 years of membership, I know too many to name individually. Thank you, AADE, for professional guidance and personal enrichment.

Dawn Satterfield has taught me about empowerment by her example. Thank you, Dawn.

Sherrye Landrum is an extraordinary editor and a true soul sister. I would not think of writing anything without her help.

Mark LeBlanc is my business advisor, mentor and friend. This book would not have happened without his urging and guidance.

Thank you, CCS Medical, for your support that made this book possible.

THE POWER TO BE WELL®

Introduction

W.C. Fields sat on his front porch one evening paging through a book. A friend came by and, amazed to see that Fields was reading the Bible, exclaimed: "Bill, I can't believe that you are reading the Bible!" To which Fields responded: "Just looking for loopholes."

How human. It is normal for people to look for loopholes, ways to get around anything that appears to be rules or requirements. Yet, it is we, in all our imperfection and humanness, who are responsible for managing our own diabetes. How do we do that?

What lies behind us and what lies before us are tiny matters compared to what lies within us.
—OLIVER WENDELL HOLMES

Each of us has a power within that guides us through challenges, inspires us to do our best and sustains us through all of life's ups and downs. I call that the Power to be Well. The focus of this book is using that power to live well with diabetes. I have had diabetes since 1957, and I have worked as a diabetes educator (actually a "life" educator) since I was the Education Director of Minnesota's American Diabetes Association affiliate in 1974. In that capacity I met many people with diabetes. Some took their diabetes in stride, learning what they needed to manage diabetes and enjoy life.

Others chose to fight diabetes or to ignore it . . . often with disastrous results.

Connecting you to your own power to live a healthier life is the goal of this book. I believe most of us who have diabetes want that goal. It isn't easy. We WANT a healthy, fulfilling life, but few of us are motivated every day to do what it takes to manage diabetes. Then, one day, we realize that diabetes is really serious and start looking for a new way to deal with it. We're tired of doing what we've always done.

This book shares some insights into how you can manage diabetes without sacrificing health or your enjoyment of life. The purpose is to connect you with your own *Power to be Well.*

In order to grow, you will need to reflect on your own life. As you read, make notes about the insights that ring true for you. Keep a notebook at hand for this purpose. Insights come through your own experiences and your intuitive, gut-level feelings. Trust what they have to tell and teach you. You already have the power to be well within you!

Personal Goals:
Set Your Own

The secret of getting ahead is getting started. The secret of getting started is breaking your complex overwhelming tasks into small, manageable tasks, and then starting on the first one.

—MARK TWAIN

The first step in the process we call the Power to be Well® is to realize that the only person who can be responsible for your health is you. The next step is to take the complex and seemingly overwhelming task of diabetes management and break it into small, doable tasks. Diabetes educators are an excellent resource to help you do this. But, while healthcare professionals can recommend treatment, the daily choices are yours to make. In this chapter you will be asked to set some goals to help you achieve greater satisfaction with your life. Life satisfaction provides the context for diabetes self-management. Life satisfaction is the why. Healthy lifestyle choices are the how.

He who has a why to live can bear almost any how.
—FRIEDRICH NIETZSCHE

Setting your own goals puts you in charge of your life. Although other people attempt to set goals for you (parents, spouse, boss, healthcare professionals), the only goal you will truly work at achieving is one you set for yourself. Begin by studying your life and discovering the goal(s) that are important to you.

Assess your satisfaction with life. Get yourself a spiral bound notebook to do the reflections that are the key to setting meaningful and realistic goals. Look at all the areas of your life and think about how satisfied you are. Consider your family life, friends, work, volunteer activities, creative activities, and what you do to take care of yourself. This will give you a clearer indication of your overall sense of well-being. A high degree of well-being allows you to live well with the challenges that life presents.

Life is not a matter of holding good cards. It's playing a poor hand well.
—ROBERT LOUIS STEVENSON

The greater your satisfaction with your life, the more resilience you have to deal with health problems like diabetes. In case you are troubled by the thought of focusing on good health when you know you already have a chronic illness, let me clarify my belief: You can have diabetes and still live a healthy life. Diabetes becomes a challenge that you can deal with—one you want to deal with because your life is so satisfying. You won't let diabetes interrupt your enjoyment of life.

Now's the time to begin studying your own life as a personal scientist with a worthy goal.

Experience is not what happens to you. It's what you do with what happens to you.

—ALDOUS HUXLEY

Take a few moments to complete the following reflection activity to help you evaluate life as you see it today.

Life Satisfaction Survey

Evaluate your satisfaction with life by responding to the following with an X under SA (Strongly Agree), A (Agree), D (Disagree), SD (Strongly Disagree).

Physical	SA	A	D	SD
I think of myself as generally healthy.				
My weight is where I want it to be.				
My exercise program is satisfactory to me.				
My eating habits are nutritionally sound.				

Psychological	SA	A	D	SD
I manage stress well.				
I am seldom depressed.				
I feel sufficiently stimulated mentally.				
Spiritual				
I am at peace with myself and the world around me.				
I can experience joy.				
I can experience love.				
I feel hopeful about the future.				
Family *(If you have no family, apply this to friends.)*				
I have close, loving family relationships.				
My family supports me.				

	SA	A	D	SD
I support the members of my family.				
Social				
I have friends in whom I can confide.				
My friends care about me.				
I give support to my friends.				
My friends support me.				
Work-related				
I am in the right job.				
I feel capable in my work.				
I feel valued for what I do.				
I look forward to going to work.				

Financial	SA	A	D	SD
I have enough money for what I need.				
I have no serious financial worries.				
I have planned for retirement.				
Personal				
I take time for myself.				
I engage in enjoyable leisure activities.				
Overall, I am satisfied with my life.				

To reach the port of heaven we must sail, sometimes with the wind and sometimes against it; but we must sail, not drift or lie at anchor.
　　　　　　　—OLIVER WENDELL HOLMES

If you feel that you are drifting or lying at anchor and you want to be sailing, reflect on what is keeping you from taking action.

Fear is a natural feeling when you are diagnosed with diabetes. You may have heard horror stories from friends or family about people who suffered every complication of diabetes. You may be fearful that those complications are in your future. First, cover your ears and don't listen to any stories that can't help you maintain a positive attitude. Then, get the facts. The results of the Diabetes Control and Complications Trial (DCCT) proved that lowering your A1c by 2% significantly prevents complications like blindness, kidney failure and nerve damage in people with type 1 diabetes. A similar study in people with type 2 diabetes, the UKPDS, showed that well managed blood glucose levels provided the same high level of prevention—and in some cases, improved the complications that had already started. Here is hope and proof that your actions can make a difference.

While these exciting studies give encouragement, there is no denying the fact that well managed diabetes takes time, effort and commitment. People sometimes feel deprived of food or forced to exercise. It's difficult to feel empowered if you feel you are being "forced" to do things. To help you succeed, keep two things in mind: 1) There is more to life than managing diabetes (review the life satisfaction survey) and 2) You make the choices. You are in control of your life.

Making healthy choices is not always easy. It can be difficult to pass up pastries or to take a walk when you don't feel like it. It might help to remember that it is the challenges in life that strengthen us. The highest level of well-being is not something we achieve *in spite of* challenges; it is something we attain *because of* them. When you work hard on your own behalf, what is the result? A surge of self-confidence . . . a true sense of *power*.

Empowerment education combines diabetes management with life management. Combining the two can lead to smooth sailing!

I am no longer afraid of storms for I am learning to sail my ship.
—Louisa May Alcott

Never lose sight of your goals for a satisfying life. An enjoyable life is made possible by well-managed diabetes.

When diabetes management becomes the focus of your life rather than something that is part of a healthy, well-rounded life, remind yourself what a healthy life is. Too often people feel they need to stop everything else until they lose weight, get their A1c down to a particular number or feel perfectly adjusted to their new life with diabetes. Actually, there is no such thing as a "perfect adjustment." Change and challenge are as much a part of diabetes as they are a normal part of life.

Life is what we make it, always has been, always will be.
                              —GRANDMA MOSES

That's why it is important to focus on happiness and fulfillment now, rather than *later*. This is well-being. Well-being encompasses all aspects of our lives, including such things as mental, social and spiritual health. It's time to consider what well-being means to you.

Place an "X" next to each statement that describes well-being for you. Feel free to write your own statements, too.

__ Having a purpose in life

__ Helping others

__ Feeling in control of life

__ Having fun

__ Believing I make a contribution

__ Feeling loved and lovable

__ Having good friends

__ Experiencing peace and joy

__ Feeling capable of handling life's ups and downs

__ Believing that life is worthwhile

__ Feeling good about who I am

__ Having hope

Many life experiences challenge our sense of well-being. If diabetes negatively impacts your health, it may also affect your well-being. Take some time for reflection now; look for insights that will help you take charge of your life.

Reflection

Keep in mind that it is both normal and healthy to experience some dissatisfaction in life. Areas of disagreement on the *Life Satisfaction Survey* provide a starting point for setting goals to help increase the level of satisfaction in your life.

Identify three statements from the *Life Satisfaction Survey* to which you responded "Strongly Disagree" or "Disagree." (Write them in your notebook.)

Why do you disagree?

How does dissatisfaction in these areas impact your diabetes management efforts?

How might your life be different if you could agree with these statements?

Action

Select one of the statements that identifies the area you are willing to focus on at this time. Write this statement as a goal:

I will include regular exercise in my life as prescribed by my healthcare team.

What small, achievable steps will you take to reach this goal? Remember to keep your steps measurable, i.e., what, how often, how much: I will **walk** (what) **Tuesday, Thursday and Saturday** (when) for **thirty minutes** (how much). Your diabetes educator can help you figure out how to increase the frequency, duration and intensity of your exercise as you grow stronger.

How much effort are you willing to put toward this goal?

On a scale from 1-10 indicate how much effort you are willing to spend on this goal.

0_____10

How confident are you that you will achieve this goal? Indicate on the scale from 1-10 how confident you are that you will reach your goal.

0_____10

Who will support you in working on this goal?

How will you reward yourself or celebrate your success when you reach this goal? Because rewards help us stay motivated, reward your behavior changes as they occur on the way to the goal. Keep your momentum going!

Barriers

Now that you've set some goals, let's look at the barriers that might prevent you from achieving them. Some personal barriers will come from the forces in your life that influence the choices you make. These forces include **family tradition**, **culture**, **advertising**, **habits**, **values** and **beliefs**. Becoming aware of these forces and their impact on you will give you the power you need to take control.

For example, a family tradition may be to snack every evening in front of the television. Might that be a barrier to diabetes management? Our culture supports fast food and all-you-can-eat restaurants. Do these types of restaurants support your nutritional goals? Advertising spreads subtle messages through pictures of beautiful women and rugged-looking men smoking. Are you affected by ads? Our daily habits such as eating from a candy dish that is out on a table at home or on a desk at work can be a barrier to real meal planning. What we value, such as the importance of eating the ethnic foods we grew up with can provide barriers to good nutrition. Our beliefs, such as "my dad died young, so will I" affect how much we will do to be healthy. Awareness of these forces and their impact on your choices will give you the power you need to take control.

Reflection

Think about the effect of family tradition, culture, advertising, habits, values and beliefs on you. Write in your notebook how you see their influence. Walk through a typical day and see yourself in situations where you encounter any of these forces. Do you see choices that are influenced by them? Would you like to make different choices the next time you're in this situation?

Action

As you identify the choices that you would like to make free of outside influences, write them in your notebook. Then you can write a focused goal to help you achieve each change that you want to experience. Remember to write your goal in small steps that can be measured. Your diabetes educator can help you set a goal that will help you take small steps toward your larger goal, but, remember, it's your goal.

Always remember that your own resolution to succeed is more important than anything else.

ABRAHAM LINCOLN

Optimism:
The Philosophy and Practice of Problem Solving

Thoughts shape both our attitudes and our behaviors. The power of thinking: "I can choose helpful and hopeful thoughts" leads naturally to a problem-solving frame of mind.

I discovered I have choices, and sometimes it's only a choice of attitude.

—ABRAHAM LINCOLN

"Reframing" is a term often used for changing one's thoughts from defeating to helpful and hopeful. In his book, *Learned Optimism*, Martin Seligman says: "Your way of explaining events to yourself determines how helpless you can become, or how energized, when you encounter the everyday setbacks as well as momentous

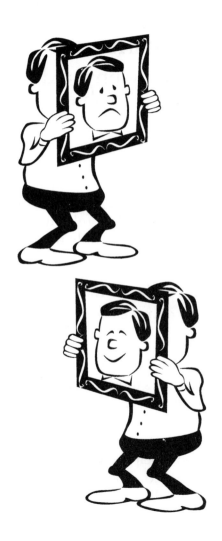

defeats." Reframing is not mindless happy talk. Your thoughts have to be accurate and believable. Dr. Seligman's research showed that "it is how you cope with negative statements that has an effect. Usually the negative beliefs that follow adversity are inaccurate. Most people catastrophize . . . Learned optimism works not through an unjustifiable positivity about the world but through the power of 'non-negative' thinking."

Compare these two thoughts about blood glucose monitoring:

1) As if age, weight, income and IQ were not enough, blood glucose monitoring provides another set of numbers by which we can be judged.

2) Blood glucose results give me important information that helps me be in control of my life with greater safety and comfort.

The first thought belongs to someone who feels like a victim. The second sounds like the thought of a knowledge-able and capable victor.

Problem solving naturally follows goal setting. Goals look easy on paper, but when you try to fit them into daily liv-ing, you often encounter problems or barriers. Barriers can keep you from accomplishing diabetes management and life enjoyment goals. These can include social events (all-you-can-eat-buffets), your thoughts and feelings (past failures at achieving goals, anger, or frustration), or lack of support from family, friends and co-workers. The classic definition of a problem is "a question raised for solu-tion." That definition takes the emotion out of the word *problem* allowing you to view the situation that has created the problem with a calmer, more logical frame of mind.

Problems are a part of life and confront everyone, everyday. Problem-solving is both philosophical and practical, a step-by-step process.

*Struggle is a decided advantage,
because it develops those qualities
which would forever lie dormant
without it.*

—NAPOLEON HILL

In this chapter, you will discover a practical, problem-solving process that you can use in all areas of your life. But your philosophy, or what you believe and think, will affect how practical it is. As you begin exploring this important life skill, take a few minutes to reflect on your goals and what you believe about them.

Becoming philosophical about life is the approach of the book, *Plato, not Prozac! Applying Eternal Wisdom to Everyday Problems* by Lou Martinoff. He says that "by getting a handle on their personal philosophies of life, sometimes with the help of the great thinkers of the past, people can build a framework for managing whatever they face and go into the next situation more solidly grounded and spiritually or philosophically whole."

To be a philosopher is not merely to have subtle thoughts, nor even to found a school . . .It is to solve some of the problems of life, not theoretically, but practically.

—HENRY DAVID THOREAU

Keep your goal in mind

Review the previous chapter and remind yourself of all the reasons you want to achieve your goals. The more important your goal is, the harder you will work at solving any problem that gets in the way. Consider, too, the reward you will have for achieving your goal.

The highest reward for a person's toil is not what they get for it, but what they become by it.

—JOHN RUSKIN

Writing about the importance of your goal will strengthen your commitment even further.

We will water the thorn for the sake of the rose.

—KANEM PROVERB

What "roses" in your life motivate you to water what appear to be thorns?

Finish this sentence:
This goal is important to me

because _____

_____

_____

Desire, determination and perseverance

You are more likely to find solutions if you have a strong desire to do so. Reflect again on why you value health and well-being. What is your "why" to live? Do some careful self-examination of your desires. Which gives you greater pay-offs—keeping your problem or finding a solution? Successful problem solving requires determination and persever-ance—never giving up.

Determination is the strength and energy you put into your efforts, while perseverance is the duration of the effort. Sir Winston Churchill, British Prime Minister during World War II, was affected by manic depression. He gave what is considered one of the world's greatest speeches to a group of school children: *"Never give up. Never give up. Never, never, never, never."*

Try again, and if that doesn't work, try again and again. Both determination and perseverance are important because we are often confronted with the same or similar problems. To keep solving them we need reinforcements: solutions to back up earlier solutions to avoid giving up.

Perseverance is not a long race; it is many short races one after another.
—WALTER ELLIOT

No one has the strength to find solutions on their own all the time without help. In upcoming chapters we examine the external and internal supports and strengths that make desire, determination and perseverance possible. With these important allies, you can turn your attention to using this practical approach to finding your own solutions.

Four-step problem solving
1. Define your problem.
Begin by stating the problem accurately and specifically. Identify the areas that are problematic in managing diabetes as well as the impact of diabetes on how you live and enjoy life. (You might list the positive effects of each action, too.)

- Sticking to a meal plan
- Exercising regularly
- Taking medication
- Managing stress
- Performing daily work
- Interacting with family
- Enjoying social life

- Experiencing an overall satisfaction with life

- Believing in future health and well-being

- Taking care of my health

- Getting support from my family and friends

2. Brainstorm and list options, things you can do about the problem.

The most effective solutions are those that come from your intuition and knowledge of your own life. In brainstorming, it is important to list as many ideas as you can without criticizing or rejecting any of them. From that list you will not only find a solution, but many solutions. It's a time for looking at your life and possibilities with new eyes.

Be careful the environment you choose for it will shape you; be careful the friends you choose for you will become like them.
— W. CLEMENT STONE

3. Take action.
Prioritize some ideas that you are willing to try. Next, choose one to start with. Write it as a goal and remember to make it both specific and measurable.

4. Evaluate.
After working on your goal for a certain amount of time—a week, a month, or a reasonable length of time—ask yourself if the problem-solving process for overcoming your barriers is working. If so, congratulate and reward yourself! If not, evaluate the goal to be sure it is realistic and applicable. It may be time to move to the second idea on your list.

"My problem is food" is not a well-defined problem. What is it about food that is problematic for you? "I eat too much" is getting closer but is still not specific enough.

A problem well-stated is a problem half-solved.
—CHARLES F. KETTERING

■ **Eating problem:** My downfall is large portion sizes and second helpings.

Options:
1) Make only enough food for single helpings (for you and the members of your family).

2) Portion out food on plates and leave serving dishes and leftovers in the kitchen.

3) Eat slowly.

Action: On two consecutive days, I tried all three options.

Evaluation: Option 2 failed because I ate the leftovers in the kitchen. Options 1 and 3 worked. My family was satisfied, and they appreciated my portioning out the food.

As one goes through life, one learns that if you don't paddle your own canoe, you don't move.
        —KATHARINE HEPBURN

■ **Monitoring problem:** I keep forgetting to monitor my blood glucose.

Options:
1) Put your meter in the kitchen so it reminds you to test at mealtimes.

2) To give more meaning to monitoring, learn how to make adjustments in food, exercise and medication dosage based on the numbers you get when you check your blood glucose. Then you can make adjustments whenever your numbers are out of range.

Action: I tried both of the options for one week.

Evaluation: They both helped me. Having the meter in front of me in the kitchen was a good reminder to monitor my blood glucose. Learning to make

adjustments in food, exercise and medication made me feel more in control. It
is easier for me to remember to monitor
when I am going to use the results to
make decisions.

■ *Exercise problem:* During the winter
months, cold temperatures, snow and ice
prevent me from doing my favorite out-
door exercise, walking.

Options:
1) Do indoor walking in the shopping
mall.

2) Join an aerobics class at the community center, school or health club.

3) Buy an exercise video and invite a
friend or neighbor to work out, too

4) Switch to indoor exercises such as stationary cycling or treadmill (all with
your doctor's OK).

Action: The aerobics class was at a time
that was inconvenient for me, and I did
not like the idea of working out in front
of my TV. I started walking a few times a

week at the indoor mall and dusted off the exercise bike that had been stored in the garage.

Evaluation: Options 1 and 4 fit my lifestyle best. Alternating exercise programs (walking and stationary cycling) brought variety to my exercise program. And, the opportunity to socialize with friends at the mall while walking is an added plus.

■ *Support problem:* Sometimes my family and friends are not supportive. (This is not well stated. What do you mean by support? What kinds of support do want from them?)

My friends and family try to tell me what to do. Not only do I not like that, I end up doing even more of what they tell me is bad for me.

Options:
1) Tell them you appreciate their concern but you don't need advice. It gets in the way of what you are trying to accomplish.

2) Let them know how they can really support you (offer to take a diabetes cooking class with you? Take walks with you? Accept you as you are and trust that you know what you're doing?)

Action: I didn't even try #1 because I figured I'd come off as being sarcastic. Option #2 worked, but it took a while. I had to explain diabetes to them so that they could understand what I was doing. Then, I told them that living well with diabetes is a lot of work, and it can be stressful. From that point it was easier to make the next point: "I really see my lifestyle as a healthy one, so if you could join me in healthy eating and getting some regular exercise that would be great support."

Evaluation: From time to time I have to point out that I take my advice from my doctor and diabetes educator who are really up on the latest treatment (without sounding sarcastic!) And, on the occasions when I do eat something sweet, I let them know: a) I compensate with insulin b) I'm having a "low" c) I allow myself to do that on special occasions, 3-4 times a year.

After you have made use of this problem solving process for a period of time, you may find it becomes automatic. You will see that problems are a normal part of life and that your skills at problem solving make you feel powerful.

If you are not yet satisfied, choose what to do next:

Check one.

___ Try another of the possible solutions.

___ Talk to your diabetes educator.

___ Talk to a friend who you believe can and will help you.

___ Other. (Describe in your own words.)

One of the things I learned the hard way was it doesn't pay to get discouraged. Keeping busy and making optimism a way of life can restore your faith in yourself.
—LUCILLE BALL

Wisdom:
How to Tap Yours

Thought and learning are of small value unless translated into action.
— WANG MING

A common expression is: "Knowledge is power." But, knowledge alone does not change behavior. There are plenty of knowledgeable people who are overweight, inactive, and unhealthy. Knowledge about the importance of good nutrition and physical activity is everywhere, easily accessed but not acted upon.

Today diabetes is considered the epidemic of our time by the Centers for Disease Control and Prevention. The epidemic is due to obesity and inactivity. Reports are found in newspapers, magazines, journals, internet articles, and news reports on television and radio that warn not only of this impending epidemic, but also the crisis that it will bring to our healthcare system, our country, and our families.

Knowledge is not power, it is only potential power that becomes real through use.
—DOROTHY RILEY

Knowledge is important but it is not enough. Once you have learned about diabetes and the healthy behaviors that help you manage it and contribute to your overall good health, then you need to tap into your inner wisdom and take action. Consider this:

I know how to monitor my blood glucose. I know how to adjust my food and exercise to keep my weight and blood glucose controlled. I know when I can handle diabetes management, and I know when I need to call my healthcare team for help. I know a lot about diabetes and good health. But, if I do not act on that knowledge, I am no better off than the person who knows nothing.

Wisdom takes knowledge to a deeper level of meaning and understanding.

In an earlier chapter, you became a scientist studying yourself. That can include monitoring your blood glucose before and after eating and exercising to see what the effect has been for you. Equally important to your health and well-being is developing a personal understanding that takes you beyond the physical to the social, psychological, emotional and spiritual realms.

Read and reflect on the following criteria of emotional maturity that was established by William C. Menninger, M.D., of the famed Menninger Clinic.

Emotional maturity is:

- the ability to deal constructively with reality

- the capacity to adapt to change

- a relative freedom from symptoms that are produced by tensions and anxieties

- the capacity to find more satisfaction in giving than in receiving

- the capacity to relate to other people in a consistent manner with mutual satisfaction and helpfulness

- the capacity to sublimate, that is, direct one's instinctive hostile energy into creative and constructive outlets

- the capacity to love[1]

Does this sound like you or someone you would like to become? Reflect on the wisdom that you have already gathered from your life's experiences. Our families are often the most influential source for the wisdom that accompanies us through life. My friend, Birgitta Rice, received this lasting wisdom from her mother.

My mother sewed all my clothes. One day she realized that the hem on the skirt she had just made was uneven. She looked at me and said, "Just walk fast and look happy." I have

[1]*Toward Understanding Human Behavior and Motivation*, Menninger Center for Applied Behavioral Science, 1985.

benefited from that wisdom in many situations and have enjoyed sharing it.

My mother was a young widow when I was diagnosed with diabetes. She didn't even know what diabetes meant. But, she had something more important than knowledge. It was wisdom, backed up with love and faith. Here is what she told me when I asked her what diabetes meant:

Diabetes means that we are going to learn so much about good nutrition! We are going to live such a healthy lifestyle that our whole family will benefit. And, you will always be a stronger, more self-disciplined person because you have diabetes.

Throughout the years as my experience with diabetes reflected my mother's wisdom, I thanked her many times. She would shun my praise by saying, "Things change." Of course, things change. From governments to fashions, *things* change, but not wisdom, love and faith.

In diabetes, much has changed. Recommendations have gone from daily foot soaks to none, and from one shot a day to multiple shots with frequent blood glucose monitoring and the use of many new kinds of diabetes pills and insulins. But the need for wisdom and inner strength, the need for personal responsibility has not changed. The power to be well has to be created new inside of each individual who is willing to take on life challenges and to seek out his or her own wisdom in the process.

Usually wisdom is woven into a story. Our stories may be quite different in circumstance and content, but the core messages unite us. One person's discovery of hope is made in a hospice while another discovers hope in a ghetto. The miracle is that different people, having diverse experiences, discover the same hope. It is in this way that we make connections with one another and with all humanity.

Dr. Rachel Naomi Remen, a physician who also lives with a chronic disease, wrote two wonderful books about wisdom: *Kitchen Table Wisdom* and *My Grandfather's Blessings*. Now may be the time to reflect on your memories of wise family members and discussions around the kitchen table or wherever these life-nourishing discussions took place. Add to this the wisdom of friends and colleagues and the people whose stories you have read.

We don't receive wisdom; we must discover it for ourselves after a journey that no one can take for us or spare us.

—Marcel Proust

Sometimes wisdom is presented in a quotation, an aphorism. Aphorisms are short statements with concentrated meaning. They are important because they take us to our own meaning, thus connecting us to our own power.

The English poet Robert Southey said: *Be brief; for it is with words as with sun-*

beams—the more they are condensed, the deeper they burn.

When thoughts go deeply into our souls, they can deliver a "wake up call" to action. Consider this thought:

Nine-tenths of wisdom is being wise in time.
—THEODORE ROOSEVELT

"People sometimes put off self-care, thinking they'll start practicing a healthier lifestyle when they retire, or when they have more time, or at the first sign of a serious problem. But sometimes that time never comes, and the first heart attack is not a wake-up call, it's the end. Are you living wisely? If not, when are you going to start?"[2]

Tomorrow is often the busiest day of the week.
—SPANISH PROVERB

---

[2] Feste, C. *365 Daily Meditations for People with Diabetes*, 2004, ADA, p. 178. Reprinted with permission.

Reflect on your favorite sources of wisdom. Books and favorite authors, sacred scriptures, people you admire, myths, fairy tales, folk tales and other stories are all ways to access inner wisdom and nourish it. Stories give us a view of other people's journeys and invite us on journeys of self-discovery. People often return refreshed, with more access to their understanding of self in relationship to the world.[3]

You might visit the 398.2 section in your local library to find traditional folktales. Prepare to stay a long time. Plan on pure delight. Discover the connections between yourself and people from every century.

Wisdom is a tree of life to those who embrace her; happy are those who hold her tightly.

—Proverbs 3:18

---

[3] Simms, L., *Becoming the World*, 2003, Mercy Corps, p. 4.

King Solomon, the wisest man who ever lived, said: *A merry heart doeth good like a medicine*, Proverbs 17:22. As you read the next chapter you will learn how modern medicine has been proving this ancient wisdom.

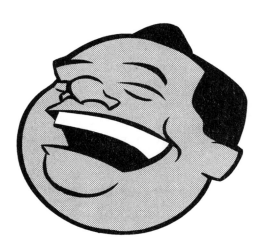

Energy:
Renew Through Stress Management

Stress does not kill us so much as ingenious adaptation to stress facilitates our survival.

—George Vaillant, MD

A most ingenious adaptation to stress comes from a highly recommended book: *Telling Tales: Storytelling in the Family* by Gail de Vos, Merle Harris and Celia Barker Lottridge. Among the delightful discoveries this book shares is research showing that people cannot recite nursery rhymes without becoming calm. They share a story about a woman in the middle of an argument with her teenaged daughter when she suddenly remembered that nursery rhymes calm you down and change your vocal tone. She began reciting: "Pat-a-cake, pat-a-cake,

Baker's man." Her startled daughter began to laugh and, with the anger gone, the two of them could have a rational discussion. Try it.

Managing daily stress is important not only for your general comfort but also in managing your diabetes. People report many different ways that their well-being suffers when they are living with unmanaged stress. Some are:

- feelings of anxiety and nervousness

- lack of interest in normally enjoyable activities

- feelings of failure as a person or any of the signs of depression

Diabetes management can suffer when people are stressed:

- attention goes to the stress and diabetes gets ignored

- coping methods may cause blood glucose problems

- stress hormones affect glucose control

- unhealthy choices create more stress

Stress is not an event. It is our perception of the event. Thoughts create feelings, and feelings can cause stress. Some people think of diabetes as their "excuse" to take better care of themselves by eating more sensibly, exercising regularly, managing stress more positively and setting an example for their family. Other people can see it as the end of life as they have enjoyed living it. Diabetes is only the "event." Your perception of diabetes and its lifestyle requirements will determine how much stress you will experience.

Since we cannot change reality, let us change the eyes which see reality.
—NIKOS KAZANTZAKIS

Talk with a trusted advisor about your feelings and the thoughts that cause them. You won't have energy to cope if you're stuck in hopeless thinking. By talking about it, you can discover why you view diabetes the way you do. Often, there is fear that a fulfilling life is no longer possible. Through ongoing education and discussion with your diabetes educator and physician and "real life experts" (the people who live successfully with diabetes and fully engage in life), you can change your thoughts from sadness to acceptance, from fear to hope. If you maintain a positive, hopeful attitude toward diabetes management, then you will see it with new eyes and diabetes will not be an overwhelming source of stress to you. Instead, diabetes becomes a series of problems to solve. The result of problem solving and coping with the accompanying stress is empowerment. When you feel in control of your life, you feel your own power.

Listen to your thoughts. Talk sense to yourself.

Dr. Seligman, author of *Learned Optimism*, said: "An individual's sense of personal control determines his fate." An outstanding example of that approach can be found in this story about Nelson Mandela. Imprisoned for 27 years, he was interviewed by a journalist on his release. The journalist asked: "How does it feel to finally be free?" Mandela's response: "I have always been free."

The greatest revolution of our generation is the discovery that human beings, by changing the inner attitudes of their minds, can change the outer aspects of their lives.
—WILLIAM JAMES

Coping is a continual process because life is ever-changing. New challenges are going to arise. Things are going to change. Even goals evolve over time. The healthy response is to be willing to keep on coping so you maintain your overall sense of well-being. That's the way to reach your goal of a fulfilling life.

The stress of life: dis-ease

Successful management of day-to-day stress is a must for everyone who wishes to live a healthy, happy life. Successful stress management is even more important for people who have a chronic disease like diabetes.

Whether it is family life, social life, or personal life, no one ever reaches a point where they are no longer confronted with challenges and stress. Stress is not only inevitable, some stress is actually essential for fulfillment. A violin provides an excellent analogy for the importance of stress in our lives. If violin strings have no stress (tension), then the violin cannot produce music. But, when too much stress is put on the violin's strings, they snap. We need to maintain balance to enjoy the symphony of life. When that balance is lost, we experience "dis-ease", which is psychological, emotional or spiritual discomfort.

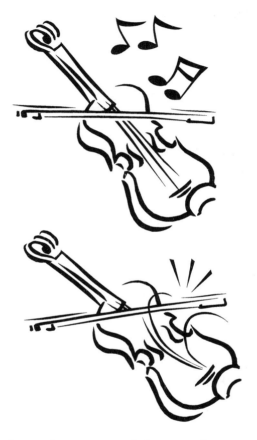

When I hear music I fear no danger;
I am invulnerable, I see no foe.
—HENRY DAVID THOREAU

The Battery Exercise

Think of your life force as a battery full of emotional, psychological and spiritual energy. The daily events of life tend to drain our battery. But, life is also the source of our energy. To prevent and manage stress, we need to assess what drains our energy and what energizes us and to make choices that keep our batteries well-charged.

In your notebook, turn to a new page and write Drains and Energizers at the top of the paper. You will be adding words or phrases under each heading as you do this exercise. Then consider which events, people, experiences, feelings, thoughts and situations drain or renew your energy.

DRAINS   **ENERGIZERS**

Look at your two lists. Do your drains and energizers balance each other? If you feel more drained than energized, what action can you take to get into balance? If any of the energy drains are problems that can be solved, try putting them through the problem solving process. Assess your thoughts toward your drains. Are your thoughts causing additional energy drain?

Do you see any stress that could be prevented? (For example, working on a project well ahead of its deadline to avoid last-minute panic and stress, saying "no" to people, blocking out time on your calendar for relaxation, or asking for help so you don't have to do it all alone?) Do you consider your methods for coping with stress to be both helpful and healthy? If not, think about the following methods and choose one to try. Then, write a goal that makes use of this coping technique to relieve your stress.

Coping Techniques

Put a checkmark by the methods you already use. Put a star by those you would be willing to try.

___ **New thoughts** help create new feelings.

___ When done regularly, **exercise** not only relieves stress, it will also prevent stressed-out feelings.

___ **Laughter** relaxes my body and brings on the release of hormones called endorphins, which are natural painkillers and spirit-boosters.

___ **Vacations** renew and recharge me.

___ **Relaxation** is a process of alternately tightening and releasing all my muscles from scalp to toes. Done with deep, slow breathing, this activity can renew my energy.

___ **Visualization** allows me to visit a favorite place for a mini-vacation. By mentally visiting a place where I have been relaxed, happy or peaceful or by imaging a place that would make me feel this way, I can regain those same feelings. Visualization can also help me work through difficult situations in a safe place.

_____ **Meditation** helps me to connect with inner wisdom.

_____ **Prayer** helps me let go of problems that are beyond human solution.

_____ Giving and receiving **support** relieves stress.

_____ **Recreational activity** both relaxes and energizes.

_____ **Talking** with friends or a trusted advisor helps relieve stress.

Add to this list whenever you find a method that works to manage or prevent stress. When you finish reading this book, assess again. If you are still feeling more drained than energized, try talking with a trusted advisor such as your diabetes educator or a member of your diabetes support group.

As a personal scientist (studying yourself, of course), you can use the world as your laboratory. In various media, you will find reports from respected studies that can give you helpful insights into how to manage stress. A study reported at a national meeting of the American College of Cardiology indicated a 22% increase in blood flow after a 15-minute episode of laughing. An additional benefit of laughter is the release of a hormone called endorphins. This hormone is the body's natural painkiller and spirit booster. Laughter renews your energy physically, mentally and spiritually. Your favorite sitcom can be good for your health, and so can friends who always make you laugh.

Humor can be dissected as a frog can, but the thing dies in the process and the innards are discouraging to any but the pure scientist.
—E.B. WHITE

Deep breathing is another well-studied and respected method for managing stress. You can add a dimension of fun by blowing bubbles. Keep a bottle of bubbles where you will see them (on your desk at work, a bookshelf or windowsill at home). Let the bottle of bubbles be your trigger to take a deep, cleansing breath.

If you let cloudy water settle, it will become clear. If you let your upset mind settle, your course will also become clear.

—BUDDHIST SAYING

As a scientist of your self, observe how you personally manage stress and ask others how they manage stress.

A woman in Dallas reported that when she is feeling overwhelmed by stress, she walks into the den in her home where she has a collection of wooden ducks on a shelf. She reports: "I receive a feeling of calm and control when I see that in at least one area of my life I have all my ducks in a row."

Humor helps.

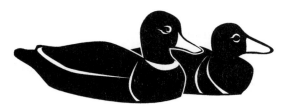

A nurse in Pennsylvania reported that there is a backroom at her clinic where she keeps a bottle of bubbles. She retreats there whenever she is feeling stressed so she can breathe deeply and blow bubbles. In addition, whenever a large carton is delivered to the clinic, the staff goes to the backroom where they put the bubble wrap on the floor and stomp on it, breaking bubbles and enjoying both laughter and activity.

A woman in Oregon uses a tabletop Zen garden to bring peace and focus to her life. As she gently rakes the sand, she feels the stress dissolve and peace takes its place.

Carrying a rubber chicken in his briefcase helps a man in Minnesota keep his sense of *humor and perspective. Sometimes he walks through an airport with the chicken's legs hanging outside his briefcase. "I enjoy the reaction of others. Their smiles, even laughter, keep my spirits up," he says.*

Enjoy doing your research!

Resilience:
Build with Reflection

Resilience is that spiritual quality that helps people bounce back when Life has laid them flat. Resilience can be described as *internal support* and defined by the word: *HOPE*. Once you have experienced the power of your internal support, you will be able to specifically define it and unendingly believe in it.

Hope is the thing with feathers that perches in the soul and sings the tune without the words and never stops at all.

—EMILY DICKINSON

What do you believe spiritual force is and what does it mean in your life? Often it is the times of greatest need that reveal the spiritual presence in our lives.

*In the depth of winter I finally
learned that within me there lay an
invincible summer.*

—ALBERT CAMUS

Sharing your thoughts and listening to others' experiences with spirituality will help you explore this beautiful and mysterious part of life. I attended a Healing & Spirituality conference at the Mind/Body Institute of Harvard Medical School. There, George Gallup, Jr., reported that the vast majority (greater than 90%) of people believe in God. Traditionally, prayer, meditation and worship nourish the spirit. How do you nourish your spirit? Consider the ways you keep your inner flame lit. It could be stories, nature, art and giving of yourself.

Stories. Once there was a man who raised butterflies as a hobby. He was so touched by the difficulties they had in emerging from the cocoon, that once, out of mistaken kindness, he split a cocoon with his thumbnail so that the tiny inmate could escape without a struggle. That butterfly was never able to use its wings. *Without struggle we remain weak.*

People. Norma and her husband, Harry, ran a hotel for years. When Harry's MS progressed to the point that he needed 24-hour nursing care, Norma ran the hotel all by herself including getting up at 5 each morning to make the pies that were served in the hotel's restaurant. Many years later, Norma was asked how she did it. With a spirit of practicality and faith she said, "On days when I was feeling down, I'd go to a movie where I could escape for a couple of hours. Feeling refreshed, I would then visit someone in a nursing home or hospital. Then, I'd get on with life."

Nature. Look closely at a pine tree. It is tall, straight, strong, resolute, yet able to bend and sway with the wind. What a lesson can be learned from this beautiful, resilient tree!

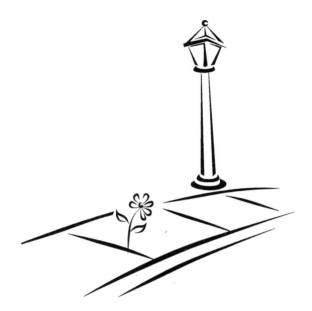

Resilience!

When a bird's nest is destroyed by a spring snow storm, the birds do not give up. They rebuild their nests using as much resilience and determination as small sticks and other building material.

Art. Art is another rich source of spiritual nourishment. Be open to receiving not only a message from works of art, but also a feeling of inspiration.

A statue of Joan of Arc in the Cathedral of Notre Dame in Paris gave me a feeling of great peace and strength in the face of great adversity and pain. Many years later I met a woman who reminded me of that work of art and its inspiring message. The woman had painful and crippling arthritis throughout her entire body. But, when I looked into her face, I never saw pain, only peace and gentle strength.

Altruism. When we give of ourselves to help others, we are engaged in what Dr. Hans Selye has called altruistic egotism. That's a fancy way of saying that we help ourselves when we help others. The spark of one spirit touching another ignites the most powerful force in the universe: Love.

Someday after mastering the winds, the tides, and gravity,

We shall harness for God the energy of Love

And then for the second time in history,

We shall have discovered Fire.
　　　　　—PIERRE TEILHARD DE CHARDIN

Rabbi Harold Kushner, author of *When Bad Things Happen to Good People*, commented that the most important ingredient in living a fulfilling life is to know that we made a difference. He said it needn't be something great. "Little deeds of loving-kindness make the difference." Rabbi Kushner suggested that just as our bodies are created to require certain kinds of food for good health, "our souls are made so certain kinds of behaviors are healthy for us and other kinds are toxic."

Theologian Paul Tillich gave us important insight when he said that God is not a benevolent cloud in the sky, separate from all of us "down here." Instead, God is as close as the closest human being is to us. Spiritual nourishment takes place whenever we say a kind word, share a beautiful thought, telephone a friend to see how she is, bring soup to a neighbor in need, spend time with a lonely or hurting person, give food, clothing, time or money to those in need, volunteer our time or talent to help others, help someone you'll probably never see again, (a stranger in a grocery store, a child thousands of miles away).

Or. . . (create your own list).

When you help others, you help yourself be stronger in body and soul. You may find that when you think of your inner power, you also think of resilience. See that overlapping as reinforcement. Your Power to be Well is surely an invincible summer, an undying song of Hope, and the center of your faith.

Within you lies abundant power to help you make it through any challenge you encounter. Find it. If you need to, get support to help you open up to it. Then, nourish it. Most importantly, believe in it. Traditional wisdom, human intuition, sacred scriptures and research findings all acknowledge the body, mind and spirit connection.

Sometimes our light goes out, but it is blown into flame by an encounter with another human being. Each of us owes the deepest thanks to those who have kindled this inner light.
—ALBERT SCHWEITZER

External Support

External support is the complement to internal support. Support is as basic a need to human beings as is a strong foundation to a tall building. Knowing that your loved ones love you is part of that support. Feeling accepted by your friends and coworkers is supportive. Knowing and interacting with others who have diabetes is a special type of support that transcends the support given by friends and family. The Greeks have a word for the quality that people with diabetes share: *noetic*, a knowing. People with diabetes understand the experience of diabetes as only a person who lives it can.

Consider joining or forming a group. You may call it a support group, a discussion group or a book club, depending on its focus. You might make up inexpensive flyers and post them in churches, libraries, community centers or work-out facilities. Announce a meeting for people who have diabetes interested in getting together to share ideas for living well and to problem solve the challenges of living with diabetes or to discuss books that have been helpful . . . whatever you wish to emphasize.

You might use the discussion questions and exercises in this book, or you may want to try a "wheel of support" as a group discussion. Ask everyone attending to bring a spiral notebook and a pen. Here are the instructions:

Draw a circle and write your name in it. Then draw lines radiating out from the circle forming "spokes" of the wheel. At the end of each line write the name of a person, an organization, or elements of your life that support you. In your notebook, describe how they support you. Once you have identified supporters and the type of support they give you, then you can evaluate how supported you feel and what you might do about it. Is your support adequate? What areas of support are missing? Where can you find that support?

Here is my wheel of support for my diabetes.

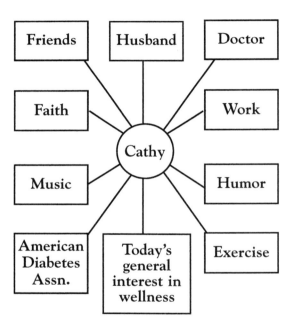

Now, draw yours!

Supporting the Group so it Supports You

The philosophy for your group can be expressed in a simple creed like this one: "We will accept one another, listen to one another, and care about one another. We will take responsibility for our own growth and continuous learning and share with the group."

Do share your stories with one another. Our stories are our legacies, not only to our family but to all whose lives we touch. The greatest inspiration can be found in stories about life. They transcend specifics like diabetes and provide power we can use for many challenges we encounter. Here is one of my favorite stories of resilience. It is a story about my father-in-law and mother-in-law.

When my father-in-law, Chris, returned from World War II, he came home to his wife, Ruth, and small daughter but no job. He wanted to be a carpenter, so he went to the carpenter's union to get permission to become a carpenter's apprentice. They told him he was too old, at age 34, to become an apprentice.

When he got home, he joined his wife at the kitchen table. He told her what happened. Then he wept. Amazed at the sight of her husband crying, Ruth reached deep inside to access her power. Recalling a favorite childhood hymn, she began to sing.

"Oh, what peace we often forfeit. Oh, what needless pain we bear, all because we do not carry everything to God in prayer."

Strengthened, she looked at Chris and said, "You go back to that union and you tell them that if you can fight for your country at age 34, you can be a carpenter's apprentice."

"Furthermore, you tell them that you are honest, hard-working and loyal and they need you!"

As of this writing, Chris has been a member of the Carpenter's Union for 60 years.

Why does anybody tell a story? It does indeed have something to do with faith, faith that the universe has meaning, that our little human lives are not irrelevant, that what we choose to say or do matters, matters cosmically.

—MADELEINE L'ENGLE

May your days be filled with storytelling, listening and laughter as you continue to tap into your **Power to be Well**.

Your power is	**P**ersonal
Fueled by	**O**ptimism
Grounded in	**W**isdom
Renewed by	**E**nergy
Sustained by	**R**esilience

End Notes

Cathy Feste is an author and speaker who knows diabetes intimately. She was diagnosed with diabetes in 1957 and began working in diabetes education in 1974. She taught her award-winning empowerment program in diabetes for the first time in 1979 and many times since then. Cathy has earned international recognition as a keynote speaker, including presentations at the World Health Organization's *Patient Education 2000* conference in Geneva and International Diabetes Federation conferences in Sydney and Paris.

Speaking to her favorite audience of people and families affected by diabetes, she has traveled throughout the United States, helping people realize the power they have to live well with diabetes and other challenges. Her work is built on the often neglected social, psychological and spiritual aspects of health and well-being. Her books include *The Physician Within* and *365 Daily Meditations for People with Diabetes*, and she co-authored *101 Tips for Coping with Diabetes*.

Cathy lives in Minnesota where she and her husband of 34 years, Dale, enjoy river boating. Their son, John, lives in Minnesota where he enjoys hunting and fishing.

Share **The Power to be Well**®, with your friends, family, healthcare team and other members of your support system: clergy, counselor, neighbors, teachers, employer or co-workers. Buy 50 copies and receive a 50% discount off the retail price. Call 800-736-7051 for special pricing on larger quantities.

Send us your comments. We'd like to hear stories about how you overcome difficulties. Share the humor, the courage and the wisdom from your life.

P.O. Box 1824
Minnetonka, MN 55345

Invite Cathy Feste to speak at your next meeting or event.

Please visit: www.cathyfeste.com